How to Give a Massage
Learning the Basics and the
Techniques of Massage Therapy

By: A.E Wilson

Copyright © 2012

Printed by: CreateSpace, Amazon. Com Company (2014)
Available on Kindle and other devices.

How to Give a Massage Learning the Basics and the Techniques of Massage Therapy

By: A.E Wilson

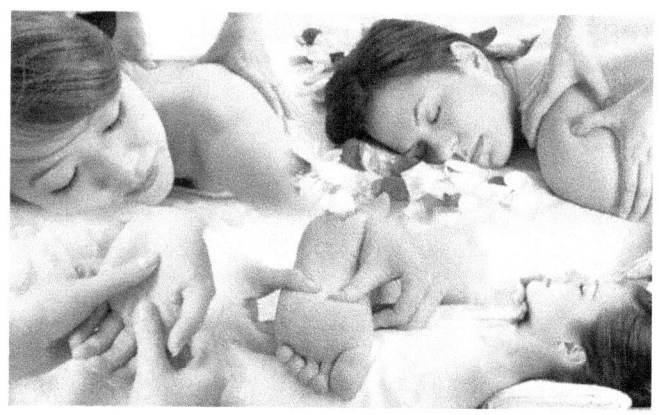

Table of Contents

Introduction

How often do you go for an hours' session with your masseuse?

Personally, I treat myself to a whole body rub with aromatherapy in my favorite spa during (or a few days after) my payday. However, that's every fifteen days only. Unfortunately, my work as a paralegal is a certain cause of daily stress and physical fatigue. Lucky me, when I get home, my husband is willing to squeeze out the strain off my muscles.

Getting a massage is not just for relaxation, though. I've learned that when my cousin tripped and fractured his leg. One of the modes of treatment recommended for him to undergo was physical therapy, which is basically massage but done by a licensed, medical practitioner.

The Science of Massage

Massage is defined as the manipulation of the various muscle layers and connective tissues of the body through various manual techniques like tapping and kneading among so many others.

Although it is not an actual mode of treating diseases, medical practitioners all over the world use massage as an adjutant therapy because it is very effective in relieving the most common symptoms. One of these is the alleviation of pain.

Today, the leaders in Medicine do not completely disregard the powers of ancient forms of treatment. Massage happens to be one of those. Now, this process is viewed as the enhancement of the bodywork's power. As I have heard my cousin's doctor say several times, massage is one of the most effective ally in a patients' healthcare and treatment plan.

Benefits of Massage

However, those aren't the only advantages of getting a 'press' work every now and then. Here are some of the unknown / unfamiliar benefits that a great massage can do for you:

- o Boost immune system by increasing the blood flow to the lymphatic regions of the body.
- o Promotes healing, e.g. regeneration of tissues.
- o Perks up one's circulation (blood) to ensure that all vital organs will get enough oxygen.
- o Relaxes, prepares and recovers tired muscles, tissues, etc. in the body.

○ Improves mood by increasing endorphins in the brain, ergo, preventing anxiety and depression.

These are the general advantages of massage therapies. Everything else will sort of follow in each of those wake.

Art of Massage

Massage has been practiced for centuries in different parts of the world. Hence, there are different kinds of massage that one can choose from today. Japan, for instance, has Shiatsu. India is well known for Ayurvedic methods. China is said to be the birthplace of Reflexology and Acupressure. It would seem that every country has its own version.

Nowadays, more kinds of massage (sometimes offered with other relaxation therapies and spa services) are being offered by various businesses. Today, more and more people opt for something that is pleasing, not just for the muscles, but for the rest of the senses as well.

Today, there are over eighty various modalities of massage. If you find that your local, favorite massage spot or spa is not offering the specific rub down that you want, go online. You will surely find that which you have been looking for or something that will interest you.

What's in the Next Chapters?

Dear Readers,

It was a bit difficult thinking about what to focus on in this 'How to Give a Massage' e-book or book. After all, there are nearly a hundred different types of massage therapies. But I don't want to bore or tire you by explaining what each of it is or by giving the advantages of every single one.

I have decided, therefore, to give you an actual step-by-step process of the five most common massages which you can easily do at home. Most concern the different body parts that are often strained while the other one is specifically made for expecting women.

Remember, it is much better to give than to receive. Besides that, knowing the intricacies of massage means that you know what is right and what you deserve when you are the one on the receiving end of the therapy.

Of course, I didn't want to leave out the other types of massages, too. So I provided a chapter just for that as well. I dedicated a section on what you need to do before, during and after the therapy so that you can get the optimum effect of massage and enjoy it to the fullest level too.

Happy reading and I truly hope that you can use some of the tips mentioned here!

Chapter I
Giving a Full Body Massage

Of all the kinds of massages offered in spa and other health spots, the most sought after is the full body rub down. If you haven't tried this yet, you should. There is something utterly soothing about this sort of therapy. Besides that, you will feel truly energized after an hour.

Sure, there are different kinds of massages (as mentioned in the first chapter). You can, of course, go and research how Shiatsu, for instance, is done and stick to that. You will need a whole lot of practice for certain types of therapeutic touch. Besides mastery, you might be required to carry a license even.

However, this specific massage that I will be describing is more of a general how-to. It is simple and easy to follow.

It All Starts with the Atmosphere

Everything about a professional massage center and spa will cater first to your senses. The room looks great, it smells wonderful; the sounds are relaxing, and so on and so forth. But you really do not have to recreate something so ostentatious in your own house.

How to Give a Massage Learning the
Basics and the Techniques of Massage
Therapy

Just make sure that the room you have chosen for the massage is comfortable and tranquil.

- o See that the room temperature is right – and that means a bit warm because the body cools down during the process.

- o The bed must be firm but comfortable to ensure right body alignment. Actually, it would be best to do the massage on the dining table – if you won't be bothering anyone else, of course.

- o Privacy is of utmost importance. Draw those curtains and close the door.

- o You can make the room feel great by adding candles, aromatic oils and playing some soothing music in the background too.

Preparing Everything that You'll Need

You'll be asking your 'client' to get rid of most of his or her clothes since this is a full body massage and you don't want to be running in and out f the room just to get stuff here and there. Everything should be close at hand.

- o Massage Oil
  Any kind of oil will do, really. However, Jojoba, Almond and Grapeseed oil are said to be very effective for this. Just make sure that you do not use anything with petroleum on it.

- o Linen and Blanket
  You do not want to mess up the whole room and have every part of it slick with oil. A plain, white, cotton linen will do. A thin blanket of the same material will be used to cover up the patient for discretion and to keep the body temperature from going too low.

- o Masseuse should also be well prepared. See that you have done your breathing exercises, taken a relaxing bath, cut your nails (very important!!!) and worn comfortable clothes.

How to Give a Massage Learning the
Basics and the Techniques of Massage
Therapy

Let Your Partner Lie on His Stomach

o   Now, let your client take his or her clothes off. If he or she does not want that, don't force the issue. It is OK if they are in their underwear. For women, unhook the bra while they are on their stomach. Remember to hook it back on when they change to supine position.

o   The client will be sandwiched in between the linen and the blanket. Except for the head, the whole body will be covered. You will only reveal the part of the body that you will be massaging then cover it back up when you are done.

Start with the Right Side of the body

It really doesn't matter which side you start. But in this case, let us start on the right side of your client. Start oiling your hand.

o   Expose the leg and the foot. Slide your hand up from the foot to the back of the knees and then down again. As you are doing this, use the tips of your fingers to knead the muscles gently.

- o Cover the legs and bare the thighs. There are three parts which you need to 'knead': the outer part, the middle and the inner side of the leg.

- o Do the same to the left side of the body. Remember to cover the right part before you move on to the left.

Position Yourself Near the Head of Your Client

- o Slide your hands from the head, running over the neck and then to the sides of the spine until the lower back. Slide your hands back up to the head.

- o As you are doing this, your hands should be moving farther from the spine in inches so that the rest of the back is being massaged too.

- o When you reach the scapula, rub around it.

- o Do the same circular motions on the shoulders. The scapula and the shoulder joints are very sensitive areas. Be sure that you massage these parts very gently.

**How to Give a Massage Learning the
Basics and the Techniques of Massage
Therapy**

o   Cover up the back once more with the blanket
and let the client turn to be on his or her
supine position (lying face upward).

Massaging On Prone Position

o   Start with the right leg once more. The two
parts which you should focus on more would
be the foot and the thighs.

Read more on the Foot Massage chapter to
know more about this. Move on to the left leg
next.

o   Cover the legs and move on to the arms. Lift
the hand up, making sure that the elbow is off
the table or bed. With your other hand, grip
the forearm sliding up to the upper parts,
touching on the biceps, triceps and shoulders
as well. Put the client's arm down and then
knead the outer part. Move on to the other
arm and do the same. Do this twice or thrice.

o   Now, take the hands and massage each as
well. Use your thumbs to do this. Start
rubbing the palms of your client, ending to
the tips of the fingers. Pull each finger,
moving it in a circular motion.

o   Finally, move back near the head so that you can start massaging the face. Another chapter is dedicated for just massaging the head and the face. You can read more about that there.

The whole session can last for thirty to forty-five minutes. But as you would notice, spas will give one complete hour for their clients. Usually, the client will sleep through this. After you are done, let him or her rest so that he or she can really relax. Give them 10 to 15 minutes for the nap and they will surely wake up totally energized.

Chapter II
Great Back Rubs

Another very common massage that people go for is the back rub or massage. Have you heard of the figurative expression 'heavy burden on one's shoulder or back'? Whatever the etymology of that is, a lot of people would agree that stress, fatigue and lack of rest are very evident in one's shoulders and back. Hence, back massages are sought-after by so many.

This is often chosen especially when you do not have enough time for the full body type. The advantage of doing a back rub is that it can be done even when sitting. The whole process can last for 10 to 15 minutes only.

Here is a basic step-by-step process on how a back massage is done:

Preparing Yourself and Your Client

Remember that massage is the most effective firm of touch therapy and a certain connection between you and your client must be established – especially if you do not know the person – so that it will be truly effective.

It is very important, therefore, that you prepare yourself well by doing breathing exercises, yoga, and taking a long, relaxing shower.

The same should be done for your client. Here is a simple run down of things which your clients should *always* have:

- o Comfort – see that everything you will be using, from blankets to pillows, addresses this need.

- o Privacy – draw the curtains. Close the door. Make sure that no one else can see your client but you, even if they are not completely naked. In this case, the client doesn't really have to get rid of their pants, only their top.

- o Treating their senses – those low-burning candles, perfumed oils wafting in the air and slow instrumentals can really do so much for your client's relaxation.

How to Give a Massage Learning the
Basics and the Techniques of Massage
Therapy

Starting the Actual Massage

Although the back rub can be done while the client is sitting on a chair, facing the backrest, the optimum effect of a massage on the back can be experienced when one is lying down.

○ As usual, spread a towel on the massage table / bed. See that you have a firm pillow to be placed under the breast bone of your client. Get ready with another sheet to be used as a blanket.
Roll a towel and position it under your forehead to ensure a good neck alignment. Another rolled towel will be placed under the ankles.

○ Position yourself near the head of your client. If you are more comfortable staying one side of the client, do so as well.

○ Rub your hands until warm. Get some pre-warmed oil and place it in the cups of your palm. Spread it all around the back in gentle strokes.

○ Extend your arms and place your hands on either side of the spine of the lower back. Press on the muscles, making circular motions while going up the shoulders. Extend your arms once more and do the same, going farther from the spine. Do this twice or thrice.

o With your thumb and forefinger, gently pinch a bit of skin and muscle, moving upwards from the waist to the shoulders.

o Next, fist your hands and use your knuckles to knead the muscles from the waist up to the shoulders. Again, remember not to put strain on the spine.

o Focus on the trapezius muscles next. This is the muscle in between the neck and the shoulder. Instead of kneading, rub these gently.

o Finally, use your palms and the tips of your fingers to gently press the muscles. Like the others, you will have to start from the lower back and move up to the trapezius muscles. Repeat this several times.

As explained earlier, and as everyone knows very well, there are just so many types of massages. This is only one type of the simplest back massages that you will encounter. As you go along, you will learn more ways on how to manipulate the muscles with your hands. For now, the methods mentioned above will surely work well.

Chapter III
Focusing on the Head and Face

Besides the back, the head and the face can also suffer from the symptoms of pain and stress. It can get even worse, actually.

If you do not get enough rest, you will surely see those lines of constant strain and worries on your face. And we do not really want to look older than we really are, right? If you do not find ways to relax your head, it is possible that you will feel more than physical aches. It will affect you at a psychological and mental level too.

Therefore, head and face massage are extremely important. Here are some of the simplest ways in which you can give your head and face a relaxing rub.

How to Give a Massage Learning the
Basics and the Techniques of Massage
Therapy

Everyday Simple Head Massage

The great thing about head massage is that it can be easily learned and you can do this any time of the day. That is, if you aren't too worried about mussing your hair up too much. Here are a couple of ways on how you can do this:

- o Shampoo motion
  Here, you are using the tips of your fingers to run over your scalp very gently, just as if you are shampooing your hair. Do this twice or thrice, ensuring that the whole expanse of your head has been covered.

- o Pulling the hair
  This is another form of head massage. Here, you will be getting locks of hair, pulling it a few times and then releasing it. You might want to start on just one section of the head so that you know where you will continue on and end.

Basic Face Reflexology

Reflexology is one of those more complicated forms of massages which you can find. This is done in three main parts of the body: the feet, hands and the face.

It is said that certain pressure points in the hands, feet or face corresponds directly to certain body parts or organs. The main aim of Reflexology is to treat specific organs in the body without using pharmaceutical or medical methodologies.

Here are some points in the face which you might want to focus on:

- o Chin
  Rubbing the indent of the chin under the lower lip with your forefinger and middle finger can help aid constipation and make your skin clearer. Massaging the jaw line, from the ear to the chin handles the sex glands.

- o Lips
  Stroking the outer line of the lower lip from edge to edge treats the pancreas. The lungs are targeted by rubbing both edges of the lip.

**How to Give a Massage Learning the
Basics and the Techniques of Massage
Therapy**

- Nose

  Your spleen is aimed at when massaging either side of the ridge under the nose. If you touch on the tip of the nose, your stomach problems will be treated.

- Cheek

  Your liver and lymphatic system problems will be dealt with if you rub under the cheekbones until the cheek joint. Digestion will be helped if you press the ridge of the cheek joint.

- Eyes

  The skin on your face, kidneys and the colon are targeted by tapping the soft skin underneath the eyes. You should start from the outside and then move in to the nose.

- Ears

  If you want whole body wellness, gently pinch the upper lobe of your ear up and down repeatedly.

- Forehead

  Massaging the edge of the forehead, near the hairline, is said to help increase your mental alertness. Touching on the center of the forehead targets the nervous system.

The great thing about these two kinds of massages is that you can do it to yourself! If you will be massaging your head, all you need to do is sit down comfortably, making sure that you are leaning at a correct angle so that your neck is well-supported.

If you are doing the face massage, try practicing in front of the mirror first. Sooner or later, you will be able to do this even when your eyes are closed.

Chapter IV
Treating Your Foot Well

Your feet are possibly the body parts which get stressed very often since these are the ones carrying the whole weight of your whole body. There are other reasons, obviously, but that is neither here nor there. The most important thing is that you do treat your feet to what it really deserves.

There are several benefits of undergoing this process. These include over all relaxation, mental and physical tranquility, homeostasis, and even sensual enjoyment. But let us not focus too much on this because this e-book is not really about that, right? It would be best if we go on directly on how this can be done.

Prepping the Feet
o   Soak your feet in warm water for about 10 minutes. You can add anything you want in the water such as baking powder and lemon or scented oils.

o   Other people choose to go for a complete foot spa.

o   Dry your feet completely with a warm, dry towel. As you are massaging a foot, see that the other is covered in the towel to keep it soft and supple.

o   Prop the legs up on a soft yet firm surface such as a massage table or low stool.

o   Spread the oil or lotion all over the foot (from ankles to toes) before you actually start.

Warm-Up

Remember, one of the most important things that you need to do is to keep the feet warm because massage can cause a decrease in body temperature. To prevent this from happening so fast, see that you 'exercise' your foot well.

o   Cup and support the heel with one hand while you pull all the toes in an upward motion.

o   Stretch the whole foot up this time and rotate it.

o   With your two hands, squeeze the foot, starting from the toes to the ankles and then back up again.

o   Place the foot back down on the surface.

How to Give a Massage Learning the
Basics and the Techniques of Massage
Therapy

Actual Massage

- o With your thumb, do downward strokes from
  the toes to the ankles. Move from the big toe
  to the smallest. Feel for those tight muscles
  and knots on the sole of your foot and gently
  loosen those.

- o Now, focus on the toes this time. Pull each
  one and then try to do circular movements for
  each. Start with the smallest toe this time.

- o With your forefinger and thumb, pinch the
  space in between each toe. Next, pinch the
  tips of the toes gently.

This is the simplest version of the foot massage but
the whole process may take about 30 to 45 minutes.
Yes, it takes nearly as long as a whole body massage,
but that is mainly because of the things that must be
done before and after the actual process.

And besides that, the actual massage is pretty
complicated. As you probably have noticed, there are
numerous techniques utilized for just one kind of
massage. Whole foot reflexology, for instance, may
take even longer than that because it is more
complex.

Chapter V
Pre-Natal Massage

To all anticipating fathers out there, listen and listen well. We have specifically created a chapter for pre-natal massage because most women will definitely need this sort of rub down (and that would be half, or more, of the total population in the world).

Besides that, this kind of massage will require gentleness, specific skill and, generally, more care, than the others. Remember that pregnancy, albeit being a normal occurrence; is a delicate condition. Utmost care must be taken.

Here is a simple run down of what happens during a pre-natal massage.

Position is Vital

Just make sure that the pregnant woman is comfortable. Make her lie on her side, sit on a sofa or cross her legs on the floor. Lying flat, supine, is not advisable because that will cause pains in her lower back.

How to Give a Massage Learning the
Basics and the Techniques of Massage
Therapy

Stick to the Lower Back

One of the reasons why you will do this massage is to alleviate the pressure on the coccyx (because of the weight in the belly). Therefore, you should focus on the alleviating the pain in the lower back. Do this by rubbing that area gently with the palm of your hand.

Feel for the spots on either side of the spine. The lymphatic fluids there may be stuck and you need to let it flow. Just roll he pads of your fingers over the area for a few minutes and you will feel the 'squishiness' get flushed off.

Loosen the Rest of the Muscles Too

Try and touch on the rest of her body as well. It might take a few more minutes, true, but that would be a few more minutes of heaven for this brave woman. Gently massage the upper back and the shoulders too.

Another area which will need attention would be her feet – especially the arches. Remember that being pregnant means extra 20 to 25 pounds in a woman's weight. And all these will be concentrated on her feet.

Take note of everything because each point in pre-natal massage is very important. Those aren't just words there. One mistake may risk the health of both the mother and her child. It would also be nice to consult with your OB-GYN and ask if your wife can actually undergo this procedure.

Chapter VI
The Basics of Other Popular Massage Therapies

Just for your information, here are some of the other well-known and sought after massage therapies nowadays. If you are in need of any of these, go and visit the closest spa or bodywork center and ask if they are offering the service that you want.

Shiatsu

This is one of the most common massage treatments made available almost anywhere nowadays. Besides the fingers, palms and knuckles of the hand, the elbows and even feet of the masseuse are being used in the process. This is said to being holistic well-being. It originates from Japan.

Swedish Massage

A lot of people have heard about this but are quite unsure what it is. Well, this type involves long, rhythmic strokes, kneading, tapping, vibration and friction. It is not just focused on loosening muscles, it also aids glandular functions.

Aromatherapy

From just the sounds of it, this is a super relaxing procedure not just for the body but also for the senses. All the oils which will be used for your massage has healing properties as well.

Deep Tissue Massage

As the name implies, this targets the most stiff and unyielding muscles and tendons found deep in the body. This is indicated for extremely rigid necks or backs, for those recovering from injuries, to relieve pain, to realign muscles and to improve posture.

Some would say that you will feel like you've been to a strenuous workout after undergoing this process. But you will soon feel good afterwards.

Thai Massage

This is another very common example of great bodywork, sometimes called Thai Yoga massage. And that is basically what it is – a combination of yoga and massage. Here, the practitioner will manipulate your body in various positions which can aid in whole body flexibility and increasing your range of motion.

How to Give a Massage Learning the
Basics and the Techniques of Massage
Therapy

Chapter VII
What to Do Pre and Post Massage

A great massage will let you relax both in body and mind. However, not all people actually get to enjoy it as much. Then they blame the masseuse for not doing their job right. Well, it could be true that it is their fault, but it is possible also that you have made some mistakes on the way as well.

Here is a list of what you should do before, during and after a massage. These tips will ensure that you really experience a good rub down every single time. Take note that all these are in the perspective of the masseuse, the person doing the massage.

List of What You Should Do Before a Massage Session

- Naked is better. Ask your client to remove his clothes, jewelry pieces and other ornaments. Tell them that the optimum effect of the massage will be achieved in this case only. If the person is a bit on the shy side, allow him or her to wear loose clothing.

  Wearing of deodorants, perfumes, cosmetics and other chemicals on the body is also a no-no before a massage.

o Try and tell them not to eat too much before the procedure.

o Don't drink alcohol or smoke also. Remember that you are undergoing the massage to detoxify.

o Soaking in a hot tub is not advisable as well. Just take a short, hot shower instead.

Things You Should Do During the Procedure

o Again, there are three things that you should have in a massage room: privacy, comfort and great treat to the senses.

o Inform your client of what you are going to do. Even if your client is falling off to sleep, it would be important that you tell them of the procedure as you are doing it.

But do not overdo with this. Other masseuses are quite talkative – and that is not at all relaxing to clients. But if they do want to talk, just let them.

How to Give a Massage Learning the
Basics and the Techniques of Massage
Therapy

What You Should Do After the Massage

- o Tell your client not to get off the massage table after the procedure. If they were relaxed enough, they would be sleeping very comfortably anyway. Just let them.

- o Drink loads of water.

- o Don't drink or smoke afterwards. It will completely wreck the purpose of the massage, which is for overall cleansing and detox.

- o Don't stay under the sun for longer periods of time after the massage. Certain oils may cause hypersensitivity reactions when in contact with the harmful rays of the sun.

- o Eat light. Go for healthier food options. Again, you have just undergone detoxification so you will be ruining the whole point of the process.

Conclusion

Both medical and non-medical experts and researchers have found out that touch has so many benefits. It does not just simply help one to relax, it can treat neurological problems, chronic diseases, alleviate signs and symptoms of various diseases and even help cure those health problems.

Bodywork definitely has become a vital part of Medicine nowadays.

This is just one of the reasons why you should go for a massage as often as you could (and can afford). But as we all know, it can get pretty expensive at times. This, now, is the reason why you should learn how to do those simple massages as well.

Try and encourage your partner or anyone in your family to learn this art and skill as well so that you, too, can enjoy the benefits of massage.

www.ingramcontent.com/pod-product-compliance
Lightning Source LLC
Chambersburg PA
CBHW070242290526
45789CB00004B/1732